HOME

REMEDIES

Inspired by

Barbara O'Neill

Teachings

A Fan-Curated Dive Into the World of

Holistic Treatments

PrimeInsight Press

Explore the entire series, available on Amazon!

Discover more extraordinary titles in the **'Get Natural with Wholesome Wisdom' collection** for a complete journey towards holistic well-being.

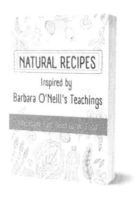

Natural Recipes Inspired by Barbara O'Neill's Teachings

Wholesome Plant-Based Yummy Food

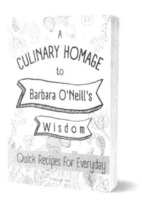

A Culinary Homage to Barbara O'Neill's Wisdom

Quick Recipes for Everyday

TABLE OF CONTENTS

INTRODUCTION

Welcome to "Home Remedies," a fascinating journey through holistic medicine guided by the wisdom of Barbara O'Neill. This book is born from the inspiration of the profound teachings of the renowned naturopath and aims to lead you into a unique and comprehensive approach to health. "Home Remedies" is much more than a simple remedy book: it is a heartfelt tribute to the teachings of Barbara O'Neill, someone we deeply admire. Inspired by her wisdom on holistic well-being, we have created this collection of natural remedies and health guidelines for everyday life.

Throughout the pages of this book, we will explore natural remedies inspired by Barbara O'Neill's teachings. Ingredients like Celtic salt, Cayenne pepper, castor oil, potato, garlic, onion, and many others become the keys to unlocking the healing power of nature. Each remedy is a testament to the holistic philosophy and the pursuit of health as an integrated process. The holistic approach considers our body as an interconnected system, where body, mind, environment, and society mutually influence each other. "Home Remedies" adopts this perspective, aiming to restore natural balance and promote profound well-being.

This book is more than an informational guide; it is an interactive companion designed to enrich your experience and put control of your health in your hands. In addition to providing valuable information on home remedies, you will find special pages inside the "Remedy Personal Diary." These pages offer you the opportunity to document your journey with each remedy, making the book a unique reflection of your individual experience. Each diary contains dedicated spaces to note the start date, quantity used, positive and negative effects, your post-use sensations, and much more. It's your personal space to track improvements, reflect on your feelings, and listen to your body! I hope you find this interactive component useful and that it enriches your journey toward a healthier and more sustainable lifestyle. Take the time to explore and note, as this diary is your trusted companion in this self-healing adventure.

Note 1:

I want to emphasize that this book is an independent creation intended solely for personal use. Our purpose is to offer an interactive and complementary experience to those who wish to explore home remedies. We strongly recommend obtaining the original copy of Barbara O'Neill's book 'Self Heal by Design' to fully leverage the valuable information provided by the author. Our book is not affiliated with or endorsed by the author or the original publisher.

Note 2:

Before making significant changes to your health, such as using herbs, altering your diet, or adjusting your lifestyle, always make sure to consult with a doctor or healthcare professional to ensure that the choices are appropriate for your specific conditions and individual needs.

NATURAL REMEDIES AND HOLISTIC HEALTH

What is Holistic Medicine?

Answering the question "What is holistic medicine?" is both simple and complex. Despite the overused and misleading use of the term in recent decades, "holistic" remains the most appropriate definition for describing a comprehensive approach to health. The holistic view considers our body as one and unique, and as such, it should be treated.

The word "holistic" was coined in the 1920s by Jan Smuts, a politician, intellectual, and philosopher, who believed that the properties of a system are not determined by the sum of its individual components, but rather the system influences the parts that constitute it.

Over the years, the development of this paradigm has multiplied, finding application today in medicine, psychology, physics, philosophy, pedagogy, and even marketing. However, the typical example of the holistic structure remains the biological organism since a living being as such should be considered a totality that cannot be expressed by the sum of its parts.

The term "holistic" comes from the Greek ὅλος, olos, meaning "totality" or "whole." In medicine, the holistic approach represents a global state of health, the union of body, mind, environment, and society where biological, psychological, and social factors are strongly interconnected.

The pursuit of health in holistic medicine is oriented towards the individual, not the disease, towards the cause that generated dysfunction, not the symptom, towards the system, not the organ, towards restoring function by stimulating the body's natural healing process (think of the cells', tissues', and organs' natural regenerative capacity). The goal of holistic medicine is not to treat a single organ or tissue but to restore balance and well-being to the individual as a whole and to re-establish harmony with the surrounding environment.

Another important aspect to highlight is prevention (also understood as a correct lifestyle), which is essential for maintaining a state of health. Each of us should have a responsible attitude aimed at preventing disease, both on the physical and mental or spiritual levels.

The holistic approach to illness means not considering the symptom of the disease but what has produced the symptom, namely the causes of the disease, which must be found in the entire, general world of the person and their relationships with the complex (the whole) of which they are a part. Once the primary cause is identified, we can treat the physical disorder from its origin rather than its manifestation.

What Does Natural Health Mean?

Natural health encompasses a set of factors such as body care, dietary attention, exercise, movement, and beauty that look to nature as an important source to draw from. When we talk about natural health, we think about how to keep the body as naturally healthy as possible, preventing rather than curing, eliminating a series of incorrect habits, and embracing others through small daily adjustments.

We are what we eat, as is clear to everyone: nutrition is the first tool that can help us heal. If we eat in a simple way, avoiding overly processed or refined products, following the rhythm of the seasons, and, as much as possible, the locality of the products, it means that our way of eating follows nature. Choosing wisely what to put on the table, listening to the body when it rejects certain foods or asks for others, means training individual sensitivity.

As important as food is movement; in this sense, efforts should be calibrated according to one's rhythms, physical structure, habit, and individual predisposition.

We are also what we think. Diseases, both physical and psychological, represent, in this journey, the manifestation of a latent demand from the body. A disorder can teach a lot; it is not just an annoyance to be eliminated as quickly as possible – one just needs to know how to listen and understand.

At the Roots of Natural Well-being.

The healing power of nature is at the base of natural remedies and so-called Natural Medicines in general. Nature must be protected in all its forms because polluted and unhealthy nature cannot heal humans. This virtuous or vicious circle exemplifies in a very simple way how crucial it is for humans to respect nature so that it can heal and save living beings. It is a simple two-way relationship, unfortunately not yet fully understood and integrated into the daily life of the individual.

Natural remedies resort to the energy of plants, minerals, water, earth, seasonality, lunar and solar flows to support humans, heal them, preserve their health, and psychophysical well-being.

Considering humans as natural beings is the first step to understanding how the laws of nature govern the rhythms of human life and must therefore be respected and followed. The human microcosm summarizes all the characteristics of the macrocosm: cellular exchanges, breathing, chemical transformations, lymphatic circulation, feminine lunar cycles, seasonal changes, day/night alternations, and the seasons of age.

Humans can be represented as a large tree, stretched between earth and sky, in constant evolution, adaptation, but also subject to disease and decay.

Today's life with its exhausting rhythms is neglecting the physiological times of humans and often tramples on them because they do not conform to mass needs.

Are you sick? Do you have the flu? Take a drug that solves your conditions quickly; in the meantime, do not stop because otherwise, you are out! This is not well-being, much less natural well-being, but it is the deleterious suppression of symptoms.

It is like disconnecting the fuse of a car that signals a malfunction. The signal is no longer visible, but the malfunction remains, and if not intervened correctly, the car will stop sooner or later. Nature and its laws, on the contrary, teach how everything is inscribed in a single life cycle, where birth and death are contemplated, growth and decay: the important thing is to be aware of one's time, which is the only precious asset that humans have and must know how to use correctly.

There is a time to play, a time to work, a time to eat, and a time to rest. The cells of the body are born, reproduce, give life to complex systems, are subject to circadian, monthly, seasonal rhythms, age, get sick, defend themselves, heal, or die. If we know how to use our body and mind well, care for them, preserve them, nourish them adequately, in harmony with their laws, which are the same as those of the great mother nature, we will know how to live our time to the fullest, in a condition of natural well-being.

REMEDIES

ONION

Onion is a treasure trove of healing properties and can be utilized in various forms: raw or cooked.

The onion (Allium cepa) is a versatile vegetable that offers several health benefits:

- Antioxidants: Onions contain antioxidants, such as quercetin, which help neutralize free radicals in the body, contributing to preventing cellular damage.
- Anti-Inflammatory: The quercetin in onions also has anti-inflammatory properties, which may help reduce inflammation in the body.
- Heart Health: Onions can help reduce the risk of heart disease by lowering blood pressure and reducing cholesterol levels.
- Immune System: Thanks to its antioxidant properties and the presence of nutrients like vitamin C, onions can support the immune system.
- Glucose Control: Some studies suggest that onions may have a positive impact on blood glucose regulation, aiding in diabetes control.

- Antibacterial Effects: Onions may have antibacterial properties and can help fight infections.
- Digestion: Onions contain dietary fiber that can support digestive health, promoting bowel regularity.
- Antitumor Properties: Some compounds in onions have been studied for their potential antitumor properties, providing possible protection against certain types of cancer.
- Antiallergic Effects: Quercetin in onions may also have antiallergic effects, helping to reduce allergy symptoms.
- Bone Health Support: Some studies indicate that onions may contribute to maintaining bone health due to their content of minerals such as calcium and phosphorus.

Using Onion for Earache

Preparation

- Steam or bake an onion until it becomes tender. The onion can remain whole, without peeling or cutting the ends to retain the juice.

Juice Extraction

- Cut the onion in half and squeeze some juice onto a teaspoon. Wait for the juice to cool slightly.

Benefit: Onion juice has healing properties that help reduce inflammation in the ear.

Application to the Affected Area

- Drop a few drops of onion juice directly into the ear, ensuring that the juice is warm but not boiling.

Benefit: The warm drops of onion juice provide immediate relief to the aching ear.

Duration and Repetition

- Repeat the process if necessary, then consider using an onion juice bandage to maintain the anti-inflammatory effect over time.

Using Onion for Earache #2

Preparation

- Steam or bake an onion until it becomes tender. The onion can remain whole, without peeling or cutting the ends to retain the juice.

Bandage Preparation

- Cut the onion in half and wrap one half in a cloth, an old towel, or a napkin. Wrap several times because the onion must be warm. Add a square of plastic to the outside of the bandage, in the part that will not come into contact with the ear; this will help retain heat longer.

Benefit: The heat from the onion promotes muscle relaxation, reducing pain and accelerating the healing process.

Application

- When the onion reaches the right temperature, not too hot (test on an arm), apply the soft part directly to the affected ear. Wrap the head and face to keep the bandage on the ear or wear a hat to keep the bandage in place on the ear.

Benefit: The heat from the onion promotes pus drainage, reducing inflammation and alleviating earache.

Duration and Repetition

- Keep the onion on the ear until it cools.
- Remove it if it cools and repeat if the earache recurs.
- Repeat the procedure until the earache is gone.

Benefit: Keeping the onion on the ear helps promote pus drainage, reducing inflammation, and alleviating earache.

Using Onion for Boils

Preparation

- Steam or bake a whole, unpeeled onion until it becomes tender.
- Let the onion cool.
   Benefits:
- Heat promotes blood circulation, helping reduce swelling and alleviate discomfort associated with boils.
- Cooked onion releases compounds that help reduce inflammation and promote healing.
- Onion heat reduces tension in the boil, speeding up the maturation and pus drainage process. Onion heat attracts pus, providing relief from pressure and promoting drainage.

Application

- Apply the cooled onion to the boil, covering it with plastic wrap or a bandage.

Duration:

- Keep the application, if possible, throughout the night.

Absorbing Bad Odors with Raw Onion

Preparation

- Place a preferably organic, raw, sliced onion on a plate in a freshly painted room or in the refrigerator.

Application

- Allow the onion to absorb any residual bad odors.

Duration and Repetition:

- Remove the onion once it has absorbed the remaining odors, remembering to address the root cause.

Benefits:

- The onion not only absorbs odors but also contributes to eliminating the root cause, providing a fresher and healthier environment. Raw onion can absorb and neutralize bad odors due to its sulfur compounds, reducing lingering odors from fresh paints or unpleasant smells in the refrigerator.

Raw Onion Poultice for Blocked Airways, Cough, Mucus, Head and Chest Colds

Preparation

- Cut an organic onion into pieces. Place the onion pieces in a plastic bag.

Application

- Place the feet of the person suffering from a strong cough and mucus into plastic bags with the onion. Secure the bag tightly around the ankle so that it remains well-sealed, then cover with socks. The onion pieces should be in contact with the sole of the foot.

Duration and Repetition:

- Keep the treatment overnight and discard it in the morning. Repeat the next night if necessary.

Benefits:

- The largest pores in our body are located on the sole of the foot. Contact with the sole promotes a reflex in the body, reducing coughing. The body will carry the beneficial effects of the onion where needed, either in the chest or head. Onion on the feet helps soothe the cough and improve sleep quality. The treatment aims to reduce irritation of the respiratory passages, offering natural relief from persistent cough. The onion emits volatile compounds that help reduce inflammation and soothe the cough.

Cough Syrup

Preparation

- Take a glass jar and place a layer of raw, sliced onion at the bottom, about half an inch.
- Add a tablespoon of honey.
- Alternate layers of onion and honey until the jar is full, always ending with a honey layer.
- Let the jar sit for 24 hours. After this time, you will see the onion floating in a syrup-like liquid.
- Filter the contents of the jar, removing the onion slices. You will obtain a genuine syrup.
- Store the jar in the refrigerator.

Application

Dosage for Children and Adults
  - For very young children, around two years old, administer half a teaspoon three times a day.
  - For older children and adults, administer one teaspoon three times a day.

Duration:

- Administer until the cough begins to diminish more and more.

Benefits:

- Onion is a natural anti-inflammatory. It promotes mucus thinning and helps clear the respiratory passages.

Remedy Personal Diary:

- *For how long have you been using the remedy?*

- *Have you noticed improvements in specific symptoms or conditions?*

- *Have you experienced any negative effects?*

- *Have you encountered difficulties in implementing the remedy?*

- *Have you integrated this remedy with other suggestions from the book?*

- *Have you consulted healthcare professionals regarding this remedy?*

Remedy Personal Diary:

- *For how long have you been using the remedy?*

- *Have you noticed improvements in specific symptoms or conditions?*

- *Have you experienced any negative effects?*

- *Have you encountered difficulties in implementing the remedy?*

- *Have you integrated this remedy with other suggestions from the book?*

- *Have you consulted healthcare professionals regarding this remedy?*

Remedy Personal Diary:

- *For how long have you been using the remedy?*

- *Have you noticed improvements in specific symptoms or conditions?*

- *Have you experienced any negative effects?*

- *Have you encountered difficulties in implementing the remedy?*

- *Have you integrated this remedy with other suggestions from the book?*

- *Have you consulted healthcare professionals regarding this remedy?*

GARLIC

Garlic (Allium sativum) possesses very powerful antibiotic properties. To make it as potent as an antibiotic, an adult should consume three raw cloves a day. For a child, it is necessary to halve the dose. Moreover, garlic is antiviral and antifungal.

Other properties of garlic:

- Heart Health: Garlic may promote heart health by reducing blood pressure and cholesterol. It can help prevent clot formation and improve blood circulation.
- Immune System: Thanks to its antimicrobial properties, garlic can support the immune system, helping prevent colds and other infections.
- Antioxidants: Garlic is rich in antioxidants that can neutralize free radicals in the body, helping prevent cellular damage and premature aging.
- Anti-Inflammatory Properties: Garlic may have anti-inflammatory effects, helping reduce inflammation in the body.
- Blood Glucose Regulation: Some studies suggest that garlic may play a role in regulating blood glucose, beneficial for those with diabetes-related issues.
- Antitumor Properties: Some research indicates that garlic may have antitumor properties and help prevent certain types of cancer.

- Digestion: Garlic can promote digestive health by stimulating the production of digestive enzymes.
- Weight Control: Some studies suggest that garlic may aid in weight control, although the effects may vary from person to person.

Flubomb - Garlic Flu Bomb for Cold, Influenza, Bronchitis, Asthma

Preparation

- Use the amount of garlic you can tolerate, half a garlic or a whole garlic.
- Crush the garlic cloves and add about a quarter teaspoon of finely grated ginger.
- Add a drop of eucalyptus oil or alternatively a drop of tea tree oil.
- Include cayenne pepper in the amount you can tolerate.
- Finish with the juice of half or a whole lemon and a teaspoon of honey.
- Mix all these ingredients in about a third of warm water.

Method of Consumption

- Drink the "FluBomb" after meals, preferably three times a day.
- Not suitable for children.

Duration of Treatment

- Generally, after the third day, there is no need for further intake.

Benefits:

- The remedy aims to harness the antibiotic properties of garlic to combat respiratory infections, improving overall health.
- The combination of garlic and ginger creates a potent remedy against cold and influenza.
- Provides relief from various respiratory disorders such as cold, flu, and sinusitis.
- The combined ingredients offer antiviral and soothing properties.
- The beverage helps reduce inflammation and alleviate infection symptoms.

Applying Garlic on Children's Feet for Cold

Preparation

- Finely slice a garlic clove.
- Place thin slices of garlic on a small piece of fabric and wrap the fabric around the garlic.

Application

- Wrap the fabric with garlic around the soles of the child's feet and cover with socks or booties.
- Remember not to directly contact the child's skin with garlic; instead, wrap the garlic in the fabric to prevent blistering on the child's foot sole, and wait for it to heal before applying another dressing.

Application Duration

- During the day, as the child plays and moves, this way, the garlic, through steps and jumps, gets crushed and penetrates better through the pores.
- Alternatively, leave the poultice overnight.

Benefits:

- Garlic, through the pores of the foot sole, penetrates inside the body and acts where it knows it needs to.
- The remedy aims to use the properties of garlic to provide natural and safe relief for children affected by a cold.
- The dressing aims to reduce coughing and improve breathing by decongesting.
- Facilitates the passage of garlic's active ingredients through the pores of the foot sole, alleviating cold symptoms.
- Provides relief from coughing and improves the child's sleep quality.

Remedy Personal Diary:

- *For how long have you been using the remedy?*

- *Have you noticed improvements in specific symptoms or conditions?*

- *Have you experienced any negative effects?*

- *Have you encountered difficulties in implementing the remedy?*

- *Have you integrated this remedy with other suggestions from the book?*

- *Have you consulted healthcare professionals regarding this remedy?*

Remedy Personal Diary:

- *For how long have you been using the remedy?*

- *Have you noticed improvements in specific symptoms or conditions?*

- *Have you experienced any negative effects?*

- *Have you encountered difficulties in implementing the remedy?*

- *Have you integrated this remedy with other suggestions from the book?*

- *Have you consulted healthcare professionals regarding this remedy?*

Remedy Personal Diary:

- *For how long have you been using the remedy?*

- *Have you noticed improvements in specific symptoms or conditions?*

- *Have you experienced any negative effects?*

- *Have you encountered difficulties in implementing the remedy?*

- *Have you integrated this remedy with other suggestions from the book?*

- *Have you consulted healthcare professionals regarding this remedy?*

GINGER

Ginger is a highly potent anti-inflammatory herb. Among its many properties, ginger is known for reducing joint inflammation. It can be used both internally and externally. Internally, it serves as an excellent anti-inflammatory and, above all, a superb anti-nausea remedy.

Other properties of ginger:

- Antioxidant Effects: The antioxidants present in ginger can help neutralize free radicals in the body, contributing to protecting cells from damage.
- Digestive Properties: Ginger can stimulate the production of digestive enzymes, promoting digestion and reducing gastrointestinal discomfort.
- Glucose Control: Some studies suggest that ginger may have a positive impact on blood glucose regulation, beneficial for those with diabetes.
- Immune System: Thanks to its antioxidant and anti-inflammatory properties, ginger can support the immune system, helping to prevent colds and infections.
- Blood Circulation: Some studies indicate that ginger may improve blood circulation and contribute to reducing blood pressure.

Ginger Tea to Reduce Internal Inflammation and Nausea

Preparation

- Grate fresh ginger and infuse it in boiling water without adding sugar.

Consumption Method

- Drink a cup of ginger tea whenever needed.

Benefits:

- Ginger, rich in anti-inflammatory properties, provides internal warmth, helping reduce inflammation.
- Reduces nausea and digestive issues, offering natural relief.
- To be consumed throughout the day to maximize benefits.

Note:
The use of ginger in everyday dishes is equally helpful, aiding during the digestion phase.

External Application of Ginger Poultice

Preparation

- Grate unpeeled ginger on a cloth or absorbent towel, creating a uniform layer.
- Place a plastic layer underneath to avoid mess.

Application

- Close the cloth, forming a square on the affected area, and wrap a bandage around.
- Secure with tape or safety pin, not too tight.
- Apply at six in the evening overnight or for up to four hours during the day.

Duration and Listening to Your Body

- Pay attention to skin reactions and heat levels during application.
- A single night may be sufficient; avoid frequent applications to prevent skin irritations.

Benefits:

- The integrated use of ginger, both internal and external, aims to reduce inflammation and improve digestion.

- The heat generated by the poultice relaxes muscles, reducing inflammation and offering pain relief.
- Ginger draws inflammation from the joint towards the skin, generating warmth.
- Attentive listening guides treatment adjustment to individual reactions.

Remedy Personal Diary:

- *For how long have you been using the remedy?*

- *Have you noticed improvements in specific symptoms or conditions?*

- *Have you experienced any negative effects?*

- *Have you encountered difficulties in implementing the remedy?*

- *Have you integrated this remedy with other suggestions from the book?*

- *Have you consulted healthcare professionals regarding this remedy?*

Remedy Personal Diary:

- *For how long have you been using the remedy?*

- *Have you noticed improvements in specific symptoms or conditions?*

- *Have you experienced any negative effects?*

- *Have you encountered difficulties in implementing the remedy?*

- *Have you integrated this remedy with other suggestions from the book?*

- *Have you consulted healthcare professionals regarding this remedy?*

Remedy Personal Diary:

- *For how long have you been using the remedy?*

- *Have you noticed improvements in specific symptoms or conditions?*

- *Have you experienced any negative effects?*

- *Have you encountered difficulties in implementing the remedy?*

- *Have you integrated this remedy with other suggestions from the book?*

- *Have you consulted healthcare professionals regarding this remedy?*

POTATO

The potato is very gentle; it heals tissues, making it suitable for application in body parts where garlic, ginger, or onion cannot be used, such as delicate areas of the body. Potatoes are rich in phosphorus and potassium, soothing reddened areas of the skin. Being alkaline, potatoes contribute to neutralizing acidity. Among its many properties is the ability to reduce and treat tissue inflammations. It can be used for sore eyes, swollen eyes, or red eyes. It is effective for ingrown nails, for a splinter that cannot be removed from the epidermal tissue. It is also excellent for sprained ankles, sprained wrists, and swollen knees due to tissue inflammation. The nature of the potato is to gently and delicately reduce inflammation.

Potato Poultice for Tissue Inflammation

Preparation

- Grate a small potato so that the poultice is not excessively wet.
- Grate the potato onto a cloth or absorbent fabric, placing a folded square of plastic wrap underneath.

Application

- Close the cloth, forming a square on the painful area, and wrap a bandage around.

- Secure with tape or a safety pin, avoiding a too-tight bandage but ensuring no leaks.

- Duration and Changing the Poultice

- Keep the poultice for several hours and change it if necessary.
- It can be kept overnight.
- Continue applying until the inflamed area has reduced inflammation.

Benefits:

- The potato poultice provides a natural remedy to reduce tissue inflammation, accelerating the healing process.
- Potatoes, alkaline and rich in potassium and phosphorus, reduce inflammation and promote the healing of surrounding tissues.
- It extracts pus and reduces inflammation, facilitating rapid healing.

Note:
The potato poultice is particularly effective for skin injuries with inflammation and can be successfully applied for several hours, promoting pain relief and healing.

Remedy Personal Diary:

- *For how long have you been using the remedy?*

- *Have you noticed improvements in specific symptoms or conditions?*

- *Have you experienced any negative effects?*

- *Have you encountered difficulties in implementing the remedy?*

- *Have you integrated this remedy with other suggestions from the book?*

- *Have you consulted healthcare professionals regarding this remedy?*

Remedy Personal Diary:

- *For how long have you been using the remedy?*

- *Have you noticed improvements in specific symptoms or conditions?*

- *Have you experienced any negative effects?*

- *Have you encountered difficulties in implementing the remedy?*

- *Have you integrated this remedy with other suggestions from the book?*

- *Have you consulted healthcare professionals regarding this remedy?*

CASTOR OIL

The use of castor oil packs for therapeutic purposes has very ancient origins, with the earliest evidence dating back to Ancient Egypt. Traditionally, castor oil packs were used for skin issues, digestive problems, and to improve blood circulation. Today, we are certain that castor oil has a significant impact on reducing inflammation in the body, it manages to penetrate deeper into our body than any other oil, promoting hormonal balance, and supporting the digestive process.

Among numerous benefits, the use of castor oil packs helps to:
- Reduce Inflammation: Castor oil helps remove excess iron from the body, significantly reducing oxidative stress and inflammation, especially in the intestines. In some cases, it may assist in reducing the size of cysts and fibroids and improving associated pain.
- Detoxify the Body: Castor oil promotes regular cleansing of the body, eliminating daily metabolites resulting from toxin processing.
- Reduce Stress and Promote Relaxation: It has been demonstrated that castor oil induces a state of relaxation and helps reduce feelings of stress. Being relaxed has numerous physiological benefits, improving the immune system and aiding digestion. Additionally, the contact of the pack with the skin produces a sense of well-being by stimulating dopamine.

- Support Digestion and Combat Constipation: The use of castor oil packs avoids the need for laxatives. Indeed, castor oil has been shown to promote bowel movements by stimulating the smooth muscle of the intestine.
- Support Liver Functions and Reduce Inflammation: Castor oil helps preserve and increase glutathione, a powerful antioxidant responsible for eliminating toxins and estrogens from the body. Moreover, castor oil is particularly beneficial for the liver.
- Promote Hormonal Balance: Castor oil supports hormonal balance, contributing to overall well-being.

Castor Oil Abdominal Wrap

Application:

1. Pour an adequate amount of castor oil onto a fabric, a large enough cloth folded onto itself.
2. Place a larger perimeter plastic under the fabric to prevent oil leaks.
3. Wait about half an hour for the oil to be absorbed.
4. Apply the wrap on the abdomen or the affected area.

Specific Benefits:

- Penetrates deeply into abdominal tissues.

- Addresses intestinal issues.
- Heals the colon, alleviating constipation and diarrhea.
- Reduces knee osteophytes without harming the bones.

Duration and Frequency:

- Leave the wrap for at least five hours a day, at least five days a week.
- Can be used overnight.
- Reusable for about a dozen times, adding oil when the fabric dries.

Generic Benefit of the Remedy:

- Contributes to the purification and healing of the abdomen, improving uterine, ovarian, and intestinal health.
- Positive impact on bone structure, reducing osteophytes.
- Part of a general well-being program.

Oil Application for Eye Problems

Application:

1. Put a drop of castor oil in the affected eye.
2. Perform the procedure in the evening before going to bed.

Specific Benefits:

- Used to reduce glaucoma and cataracts before surgery.
- Attracts and removes unwanted particles in the eye.
- Relieves tired eyes in the evening.

Duration and Frequency:

- Apply a drop to each eye in the evening before going to bed.

Generic Benefit of the Remedy:

- Contributes to the relief and maintenance of eye health.
- Natural support practice before necessary surgeries.

Reduction of Joint Inflammation with Castor Oil

Application:

1. Soak a cloth or gauze with castor oil.
2. Perform the procedure as in remedy number 14.
3. Wrap the fabric around the affected area (knees or elbows).

Specific Benefits:

- Reduction of joint inflammation and swelling.

Duration and Frequency:

- Apply the castor oil wrap for at least five hours a day, at least five days a week.

Generic Benefit of the Remedy:

- Promotes joint mobility.
- Contributes to reducing pain associated with inflammatory joint conditions.

Remedy Personal Diary:

- *For how long have you been using the remedy?*

- *Have you noticed improvements in specific symptoms or conditions?*

- *Have you experienced any negative effects?*

- *Have you encountered difficulties in implementing the remedy?*

- *Have you integrated this remedy with other suggestions from the book?*

- *Have you consulted healthcare professionals regarding this remedy?*

Remedy Personal Diary:

- *For how long have you been using the remedy?*

- *Have you noticed improvements in specific symptoms or conditions?*

- *Have you experienced any negative effects?*

- *Have you encountered difficulties in implementing the remedy?*

- *Have you integrated this remedy with other suggestions from the book?*

- *Have you consulted healthcare professionals regarding this remedy?*

Remedy Personal Diary:

- *For how long have you been using the remedy?*

- *Have you noticed improvements in specific symptoms or conditions?*

- *Have you experienced any negative effects?*

- *Have you encountered difficulties in implementing the remedy?*

- *Have you integrated this remedy with other suggestions from the book?*

- *Have you consulted healthcare professionals regarding this remedy?*

CHARCOAL

Activated charcoal, or activated carbon, is known for some therapeutic properties, especially in the field of detoxification and the treatment of poisonings. However, it's important to emphasize that activated charcoal is not suitable for all medical situations, and its use must be approached with caution.

Here are some therapeutic properties associated with activated charcoal:

- Toxin Absorption: Activated charcoal has a porous structure that allows it to absorb toxic substances and poisons in the gastrointestinal tract. For this reason, it is often used as a remedy in cases of poisoning or ingestion of harmful substances.
- Detoxification: Activated charcoal can be used as part of detox programs to help remove harmful substances from the body. However, it's important to use it under the supervision of a healthcare professional.
- Gas and Bloating: It can help reduce intestinal gas and bloating by absorbing gases produced during digestion.
- Digestive Support: In some cases, activated charcoal can be used to alleviate symptoms of indigestion and gastrointestinal discomfort.
- Body Odors and Bad Breath: Activated charcoal can help reduce body odors and bad breath by absorbing the substances responsible for these odors.

- Digestive Irregularities: It can be used to help regulate bowel movements in cases of diarrhea or constipation, but its effectiveness may vary.
- Skin Support: It can be used in face masks or soaps to help absorb impurities and excess oil from the skin.

It's crucial to note that activated charcoal can interfere with the absorption of certain medications and nutrients, so it's important to consult with a healthcare professional before using it, especially if you are taking medications or have specific medical conditions. Improper use of activated charcoal can pose risks, and it should always be used according to the guidance of an expert.

Internal Application of Charcoal for Poison Ingestion

Preparation:

- Activated charcoal can be in the form of tablets or powder.
- Mix 1-2 teaspoons of charcoal powder in a glass of water.

Intake:
- Drink the solution as quickly as possible.

Duration:

- Can be taken immediately after ingesting poison.

Benefits:

- Charcoal absorbs and neutralizes poisons in the digestive tract.
- Provides rapid relief from poisoning symptoms.

Internal Application of Charcoal for Gastric Disturbances, Diarrhea, or Bloating

Preparation:

- Activated charcoal can be in the form of tablets or powder.
- Mix 1-2 teaspoons of charcoal powder in water.

Intake:

- Consume after meals or when experiencing symptoms of gastric disturbances.

Duration:
- Can be taken regularly to treat gastric disturbances or diarrhea.

Benefits:

- Charcoal absorbs toxins in the stomach, reducing gastric disturbances, diarrhea, and bloating.
- Promotes better digestion.

External Application of Charcoal for Insect and Spider Bites

Preparation:

- Mix charcoal powder with flour or cooked flax seeds to form a paste, adding enough water.

Application:

- Apply the paste to the area affected by bee, wasp, or ant stings.

Duration:

- Leave on for at least 20-30 minutes.

Benefits:

- Charcoal neutralizes the venom from stings, reducing swelling and pain.
- Provides immediate relief.

External Application of Charcoal for Wounds, Boils, or Ingrown Nails

Preparation:

- Mix charcoal with ground and cooked flax seeds to form a paste, adding water and mixing well.

Application:

- Apply the paste to the wound or boil.
- Cover with a bandage and leave on for at least 1-2 hours or overnight.

Benefits:

- Charcoal helps prevent infections, accelerating the healing process of wounds and boils.
- Reduces pain and swelling.

Remedy Personal Diary:

- *For how long have you been using the remedy?*

- *Have you noticed improvements in specific symptoms or conditions?*

- *Have you experienced any negative effects?*

- *Have you encountered difficulties in implementing the remedy?*

- *Have you integrated this remedy with other suggestions from the book?*

- *Have you consulted healthcare professionals regarding this remedy?*

Remedy Personal Diary:

- *For how long have you been using the remedy?*

- *Have you noticed improvements in specific symptoms or conditions?*

- *Have you experienced any negative effects?*

- *Have you encountered difficulties in implementing the remedy?*

- *Have you integrated this remedy with other suggestions from the book?*

- *Have you consulted healthcare professionals regarding this remedy?*

Remedy Personal Diary:

- *For how long have you been using the remedy?*

- *Have you noticed improvements in specific symptoms or conditions?*

- *Have you experienced any negative effects?*

- *Have you encountered difficulties in implementing the remedy?*

- *Have you integrated this remedy with other suggestions from the book?*

- *Have you consulted healthcare professionals regarding this remedy?*

RED ELM

Red elm, scientifically known as Ulmus rubra, is a plant traditionally used in some cultures for its alleged therapeutic properties. However, it's important to note that many of the claims regarding the healing properties of red elm are not supported by robust scientific evidence.

Therapeutic properties of red elm:

- Anti-Inflammatory Effect: Red elm is believed to have anti-inflammatory properties and has been traditionally used to alleviate inflammatory conditions such as sore throat, cough, and skin irritations.
- Digestive System Support: In some traditions, red elm has been used to treat gastrointestinal disorders like diarrhea. It is thought to form a protective layer on the gastric mucosa.
- Potential Diuretic Effect: Some believe that red elm may have a diuretic effect, aiding in the elimination of excess fluids from the body.
- Skin Support: Traditionally, red elm has been used externally to relieve skin irritations, burns, and rashes.
- Respiratory Benefits: Red elm is believed to have respiratory benefits, and certain preparations from this plant are used to soothe coughs and sore throats.

- Antioxidant Effect: Some preliminary studies suggest that red elm might have antioxidant properties, which could help counteract oxidative stress in the body.

Drinking Red Elm

Preparation:

- Put a teaspoon of red elm in half a glass of water.
- Stir quickly and well to avoid the formation of gelatin.

Application:

- Drink immediately after preparation, as it may become too thick otherwise.

Benefits:

- Growth stimulant for healing the gastrointestinal tract.
- Useful for resolving diarrhea or stomach pain.

Red Elm and Charcoal Poultice for Bee Stings, Insect Bites, or Snake Bites

Preparation:

- Combine a teaspoon of red elm and a teaspoon of activated charcoal in a bowl.
- Add some water to achieve a gelatinous consistency.
- Stir well until a gel-like compound is obtained.
- Spread the poultice on a cloth or absorbent towel, under which a larger plastic square is placed.

Application:

- Apply to the affected area for several hours or overnight.
- Can be used on bee stings, insect bites, snake bites, sore eyes, boils, or swelling situations.

Benefits:

- Absorbs and neutralizes poisons.
- Provides immediate relief from insect bites.

Remedy Personal Diary:

- *For how long have you been using the remedy?*

- *Have you noticed improvements in specific symptoms or conditions?*

- *Have you experienced any negative effects?*

- *Have you encountered difficulties in implementing the remedy?*

- *Have you integrated this remedy with other suggestions from the book?*

- *Have you consulted healthcare professionals regarding this remedy?*

Remedy Personal Diary:

- *For how long have you been using the remedy?*

- *Have you noticed improvements in specific symptoms or conditions?*

- *Have you experienced any negative effects?*

- *Have you encountered difficulties in implementing the remedy?*

- *Have you integrated this remedy with other suggestions from the book?*

- *Have you consulted healthcare professionals regarding this remedy?*

CAYENNE PEPPER

Cayenne pepper is a plant and comes from the Solanaceae family, it is rich in piperine and antioxidants, and is known for its digestive stimulating properties. Consumed internally, it facilitates digestion, it is also. Used to improve circulation and combat gastric ulcers. Applied externally, black pepper is used in poultices to promote wound healing. Awaken body parts such as limbs and thyroid.

Cayenne pepper, also known as Capsicum annuum or Cayenne chili, is a spicy spice derived from red peppers. This pepper contains a substance called capsaicin, responsible for its spicy flavor and associated with various healing properties.

Healing properties of cayenne pepper:

- Anti-Inflammatory Effect: The capsaicin in cayenne pepper is known for its anti-inflammatory properties. It can be used topically in creams or ointments to alleviate inflammation associated with conditions such as arthritis.
- Pain Relief: Capsaicin can act as a topical analgesic, reducing the perception of pain. It is often used to relieve muscle, joint, and neuropathic pain.
- Improved Blood Circulation: Capsaicin may contribute to improving blood circulation by stimulating blood vessels and reducing blood pressure.
- Digestive Support: Cayenne pepper may have positive effects on digestion by stimulating saliva and gastric fluid production. It can also act as a mild laxative.

- Antioxidant Properties: Capsaicin is an antioxidant, helping to neutralize free radicals in the body and contributing to overall health.
- Thermogenic Effect: Capsaicin can increase thermogenesis, the production of heat in the body, potentially contributing to weight loss. However, effects may vary and should be part of a comprehensive approach to weight management.
- Reduced Cold Symptoms: Cayenne pepper's ability to stimulate sweating can help reduce cold symptoms such as congestion and fever.
- Possible Heart Health Support: Some studies indicate that capsaicin may have positive effects on heart health, helping to lower cholesterol levels and improve heart function.

Cayenne Pepper Wrap for Rejuvenating Circulation and Addressing Numbness and Cold Feet

Preparation:

- Lay a piece of plastic wrap on a hard surface.
- Horizontally, place a folded kitchen paper sheet and lightly spray oil on it.
- Sprinkle half a teaspoon of cayenne pepper on the paper.

Application:

Place the cold or numb foot on the cayenne pepper.

Wrap the foot with plastic wrap and wear a sock.

Duration:

Leave the wrap overnight. If there is numbness, repeat for two non-consecutive nights.

Benefits:

- Rejuvenates circulation in areas with poor sensitivity or coldness.
- Addresses numbness over multiple sessions.

Cayenne Pepper Wrap for Those with Hypothyroidism

Preparation:

Spread a rectangle of plastic wrap on a hard surface.

In the center, place a small piece of folded kitchen paper, wet with a few drops of oil to fix the cayenne pepper.

Sprinkle a modest amount of pepper, less than half a teaspoon.

Application:

- Place the wrap at the base of the neck, on the thyroid gland, securing the wrap behind the neck so that it doesn't slip.

Duration:

- Keep the wrap for a few hours, preferably in the morning.

Benefits:

- Draws blood to the thyroid gland to stimulate it.

Note:
Intense physical activity further contributes to maintaining thyroid balance.

In the world of wellness and health, the controversy surrounding cayenne pepper is at the center of debate. Some doctors liken it to common chili, raising concerns about heating the stomach. This raises questions about opinions on cayenne pepper and its authenticity.

Drawing on Jethro Claus's book "Back to Eden," we can highlight the effectiveness of cayenne pepper as a blood flow stimulant without acting as a nervous stimulant. Cayenne pepper, known as Capsicum annuum, is considered a fundamental blood stimulant, enhancer of other herbs, and to ensure its quality, it is necessary to purchase it from specialized herb companies to ensure freshness. Bright red color indicates freshness, while brown indicates aging.

Remedy Personal Diary:

- *For how long have you been using the remedy?*

- *Have you noticed improvements in specific symptoms or conditions?*

- *Have you experienced any negative effects?*

- *Have you encountered difficulties in implementing the remedy?*

- *Have you integrated this remedy with other suggestions from the book?*

- *Have you consulted healthcare professionals regarding this remedy?*

Remedy Personal Diary:

- *For how long have you been using the remedy?*

- *Have you noticed improvements in specific symptoms or conditions?*

- *Have you experienced any negative effects?*

- *Have you encountered difficulties in implementing the remedy?*

- *Have you integrated this remedy with other suggestions from the book?*

- *Have you consulted healthcare professionals regarding this remedy?*

CABBAGE

Cabbage, intended as a food, has many healing properties for humans:

- Antioxidant: Cabbage is rich in antioxidants such as vitamin C and flavonoids, which help counteract free radicals in the body and protect cells from damage.
- Anti-Inflammatory: Compounds in cabbage, especially those from the glucosinolate family, have demonstrated anti-inflammatory properties that may contribute to reducing inflammation in the body.
- Digestive Support: Cabbage is a good source of fiber, promoting digestive system health. Fiber aids in intestinal regularity and can be helpful in preventing constipation.
- Cholesterol Reduction: Some studies suggest that regular consumption of cabbage may contribute to lowering cholesterol levels in the blood, thanks to the presence of fiber and phytosterols.
- Cardiovascular Health Benefits: In addition to cholesterol reduction, cabbage can support cardiovascular health through its content of antioxidants and phytochemicals that promote blood vessel health.
- Detox: Cabbage contains compounds like glucosinolates that can support the liver's detoxification phase, helping the body eliminate harmful substances.
- Antiulcer Properties: Some studies suggest that cabbage may have protective effects against gastric ulcers, in part

due to its ability to stimulate mucous production in the stomach.

- Weight Management: Cabbage is a low-calorie food, rich in fiber and nutrients. Its consumption can contribute to a balanced diet and weight management.
- Anti-Cancer Properties: Some phytochemical compounds in cabbage, such as glucosinolates, have been studied for their potential role in cancer prevention.
- Immune Support: The presence of vitamin C in cabbage can contribute to supporting the immune system, helping the body defend against infections and diseases.

But cabbage is renowned for its anti-inflammatory properties for external use. Applying the leaves to the skin can help reduce swelling and relieve pain. This method is commonly used to manage breast swelling during breastfeeding and can be adapted to other inflammatory situations.

In fact the proposed remedy is an external application of cabbage.

Therapeutic Application of Cabbage to Reduce Inflammation and Swelling

Preparation:

Cabbage, a versatile vegetable, can be utilized to address tissue inflammations. To create a cabbage compress, one can use raw leaves or make them more flexible by either soaking them in boiling water or pounding them with a meat tenderizer.

Application:

Apply the cabbage compress directly to the inflamed area. For instance, in the case of swollen and painful breasts during breastfeeding, cabbage leaves can be placed inside the bra. Similarly, in the case of ankle sprains, cabbage leaves can be wrapped around the inflamed area.

Duration:

The duration of the application varies depending on the severity of the inflammation. Cabbage leaves can be left in place until significant relief is felt. In the context of breastfeeding, the leaves can be replaced as they dry out.

Notes:

Cabbage leaves have found application in maternity hospital settings in Australia and the United States. However, it is crucial to discuss the use of natural remedies, including cabbage, with a healthcare professional, especially in more severe or persistent situations.

Remedy Personal Diary:

- *For how long have you been using the remedy?*

- *Have you noticed improvements in specific symptoms or conditions?*

- *Have you experienced any negative effects?*

- *Have you encountered difficulties in implementing the remedy?*

- *Have you integrated this remedy with other suggestions from the book?*

- *Have you consulted healthcare professionals regarding this remedy?*

Remedy Personal Diary:

- *For how long have you been using the remedy?*

- *Have you noticed improvements in specific symptoms or conditions?*

- *Have you experienced any negative effects?*

- *Have you encountered difficulties in implementing the remedy?*

- *Have you integrated this remedy with other suggestions from the book?*

- *Have you consulted healthcare professionals regarding this remedy?*

ALOE VERA

Succulent plant used since ancient times for its numerous properties.

Properties of Aloe Vera for External Use:

- Skin Hydration: Aloe vera is rich in water and helps moisturize the skin, making it beneficial for individuals with dry skin.
- Soothing and Calming: Aloe vera has soothing and calming properties that can help reduce skin irritation and redness, especially in the case of sunburn or irritated skin.
- Wound Healing: Aloe vera can contribute to the wound healing process, accelerating the regeneration of skin cells.
- Sunburn Relief: Applying aloe vera gel can provide immediate relief for sunburn, reducing pain and promoting healing.
- Acne Treatment: Aloe vera can be used to reduce acne inflammation and promote the healing of pimples.
- Antibacterial and Antifungal: Thanks to its antibacterial and antifungal properties, aloe vera can be used to treat minor skin infections or fungi.
- Anti-Aging: Aloe vera contains antioxidants and can help reduce signs of aging, such as wrinkles and fine lines, keeping the skin elastic.
- Skin Brightening: Applying aloe vera gel can give the skin a brighter and fresher appearance.

- Relief for Itching and Skin Allergies: Aloe vera can reduce itching and provide relief for skin irritations caused by allergies or dermatitis.
- Skin Sanitization: The antibacterial properties of aloe vera can help keep the skin clean and protect it from infections.

Utilizing Aloe Vera to Expedite Burn Healing

Preparation and Application:

To harness the healing power of aloe vera for burns, cut a leaf in half and apply the soothing gel directly to the affected area, even in cases of significant skin damage.

Benefits:

Aloe vera's healing properties, combined with its growth-stimulating attributes, can significantly contribute to skin regeneration and hasten the recovery process. The natural emollient found in aloe vera offers soothing relief to damaged skin.

Note:
While the use of aloe vera for burn treatment is a time-tested and recognized practice, individual skin reactions should be monitored. In cases of severe burns or injuries, seeking medical advice is crucial for appropriate care.

Remedy Personal Diary:

- *For how long have you been using the remedy?*

- *Have you noticed improvements in specific symptoms or conditions?*

- *Have you experienced any negative effects?*

- *Have you encountered difficulties in implementing the remedy?*

- *Have you integrated this remedy with other suggestions from the book?*

- *Have you consulted healthcare professionals regarding this remedy?*

Remedy Personal Diary:

- *For how long have you been using the remedy?*

- *Have you noticed improvements in specific symptoms or conditions?*

- *Have you experienced any negative effects?*

- *Have you encountered difficulties in implementing the remedy?*

- *Have you integrated this remedy with other suggestions from the book?*

- *Have you consulted healthcare professionals regarding this remedy?*

EPSOM SALT

Epsom salt, scientifically known as magnesium sulfate, is a chemical compound made up of magnesium, sulfur and oxygen. It appears as colorless or white crystals, and is known for its therapeutic and beneficial properties.

The name "Epsom" comes from the town of Epsom in England, where it was first discovered and where it was extracted naturally from saline springs.

Epsom salt is widely used for therapeutic purposes, these are its main properties:

- Stress Reduction: Epsom salt baths can help reduce stress and promote muscle relaxation, thanks to the presence of magnesium.
- Muscle Pain Relief: Epsom salt can be used to alleviate muscle aches and tension. Magnesium contributes to muscle relaxation.
- Relief for Sprains and Bruises: Applied topically, Epsom salt can help reduce swelling, sprains, and bruises.
- Skin Exfoliation: Mixed with oil or water, Epsom salt can be used as a scrub to exfoliate the skin, removing dead cells and improving texture.
- Natural Laxative: Taken orally under medical supervision, Epsom salt can act as a natural laxative to relieve constipation.

- Sleep Improvement: Taking an Epsom salt bath before bedtime can contribute to better sleep quality due to its relaxing effects.
- Nail and Skin Support: Epsom salt can be used to strengthen nails and promote skin health, especially in solutions or baths.
- Reduction of Swelling: Epsom salt baths can help reduce swelling in the feet and ankles.
- Scalp Detox: Mixed with shampoo, Epsom salt can be used as a scalp scrub to remove excess sebum and dead cells.

Epsom Salt for Muscle Relaxation, Insomnia Relief, and Stress Alleviation

Preparation:

Before bedtime, prepare a warm bath by adding two cups of Epsom salt. Epsom salt, rich in magnesium, is used in hot baths to relax muscles, alleviate stress, and promote sleep.

Benefits:

Acts as a natural muscle relaxant. Magnesium and moisture relax muscles, providing relief for various muscular and mental conditions.

Epsom Salt Treatment for Burns

Preparation and Description:

Take a container filled halfway with water. Add a tablespoon of Epsom salt and mix until a saturated solution is achieved. Immerse the burned body part in the solution or apply a wet compress to the affected area.

Benefits:

Effectively treats burns, facilitates healing, and reduces pain. The use of an infused compress can significantly alleviate long-term pain.

Note:
In all cases, it is advisable to consult a healthcare professional, especially in more severe or persistent situations.

Iodine Deficiency Test

Preparation:
Purchase iodine from a pharmacy. Make a mark on the side of the arm with iodine, creating a brown stain. Observe how long the stain lasts. If the iodine mark disappears within an hour, it may indicate iodine deficiency.

Benefits:
Provides a quick indicator of iodine availability in the body, crucial for thyroid health.

How to Increase Iodine Levels and Support Thyroid Function

Description:
Iodine is vital for the thyroid. To address iodine deficiency, it is helpful to remove mercury fillings, as mercury absorbs the selenium necessary for converting iodine into thyroxine. The deficiency can be compensated by consuming 5 Brazilian nuts until selenium levels are sufficient for proper thyroid function.

Benefits:
Ensures proper thyroid function and provides practical alternatives to obtain sufficient iodine.

Remedy Personal Diary:

- *For how long have you been using the remedy?*

- *Have you noticed improvements in specific symptoms or conditions?*

- *Have you experienced any negative effects?*

- *Have you encountered difficulties in implementing the remedy?*

- *Have you integrated this remedy with other suggestions from the book?*

- *Have you consulted healthcare professionals regarding this remedy?*

Remedy Personal Diary:

- *For how long have you been using the remedy?*

- *Have you noticed improvements in specific symptoms or conditions?*

- *Have you experienced any negative effects?*

- *Have you encountered difficulties in implementing the remedy?*

- *Have you integrated this remedy with other suggestions from the book?*

- *Have you consulted healthcare professionals regarding this remedy?*

Hydrotherapy Treatment for Headaches

Description:

Prepare a basin and a kettle of water. Heat the water and keep the kettle filled and ready for use.

Application:

Immerse your feet in the basin filled with warm water and keep them in the warm water for about 20 minutes, ensuring the water stays consistently warm and doesn't cool down.

Benefits:

The warm foot bath aids in relieving headaches, even those related to caffeine withdrawal. It helps decongest blood flow to the head, subsequently reducing pain.

Remedy for Swollen Legs and Water Retention #1

Preparation:

Obtain Celtic or Himalayan salt crystals. Increase your daily water intake to at least 2 liters of water per day.

Application:

Before drinking a glass of water, place a whole salt crystal on your tongue and then drink. Remember to sip water in small amounts very frequently throughout the day.

Benefits:

The salt crystal aids water absorption by cells, helping replenish water dispersed from the body during the day. It assists in reducing leg swelling.

Remedy for Swollen Legs and Water Retention #2

Preparation:

Prepare or have your trusted herbalist prepare a tea containing celery, parsley, and couch grass.

Application:

Drink one liter of this tea every day until water retention reduces, and the legs de-swell.

Benefits:

The herbs in the tea help the kidneys function well, aiding in eliminating water retention. Regular consumption gradually reduces leg swelling, especially when accompanied by a plant-based diet rich in leafy green vegetables.

Hot-Cold Hydrotherapy

Hot-cold hydrotherapy provides a dynamic approach to improve circulation and alleviate swelling, particularly useful in the case of localized injuries or inflammation.

Procedure

 - Take two containers with water, one hot and the other cold with ice cubes.
 - Alternate immersion: 3 minutes in hot water and 30 seconds in cold water, repeated for 3 cycles.
 - Perform hydrotherapy every two hours or at least 3 times a day.

Benefits:

 - Stimulation of blood circulation.
 - Reduction of swelling.
 - Pain relief.

Remedy Personal Diary:

- *For how long have you been using the remedy?*

- *Have you noticed improvements in specific symptoms or conditions?*

- *Have you experienced any negative effects?*

- *Have you encountered difficulties in implementing the remedy?*

- *Have you integrated this remedy with other suggestions from the book?*

- *Have you consulted healthcare professionals regarding this remedy?*

Remedy Personal Diary:

- *For how long have you been using the remedy?*

- *Have you noticed improvements in specific symptoms or conditions?*

- *Have you experienced any negative effects?*

- *Have you encountered difficulties in implementing the remedy?*

- *Have you integrated this remedy with other suggestions from the book?*

- *Have you consulted healthcare professionals regarding this remedy?*

Remedy Personal Diary:

- *For how long have you been using the remedy?*

- *Have you noticed improvements in specific symptoms or conditions?*

- *Have you experienced any negative effects?*

- *Have you encountered difficulties in implementing the remedy?*

- *Have you integrated this remedy with other suggestions from the book?*

- *Have you consulted healthcare professionals regarding this remedy?*

Gratitude and Blessing of the Poultice

- Conclude the treatment by expressing gratitude for the used poultice contributes to mental and physical well-being.

- Offer a prayer or request a divine blessing for the poultice and the treatment process. Prayer can be a moment of spiritual connection, contributing to the success of the treatment.

- Pay attention to body reactions during poultice application, adapting the treatment as needed. Attentive listening guides treatment adjustment to individual reactions.

- Recognize any improvements or feelings of relief resulting from poultice use. Recognizing positive results contributes to maintaining a positive attitude towards the treatment.

The approach of gratitude, blessing, and attentive listening, combined with the use of natural remedies, aims to enhance overall well-being, both physically and spiritually.

SPECIFIC ORGAN TREATMENTS

FOR A HEALTHY COLON

The colon is the terminal portion of our intestines, where digestion residues arrive. Here, the absorption of water and minerals occurs, promoting the formation and evacuation of feces. The colon is characterized by a rich bacterial flora (intestinal microbiota), playing a crucial role both in intestinal health and the overall well-being of the body.

Colon Stimulation

Physical Exercise:

> Particularly effective is pilates, which gently massages the colon. It is recommended to dedicate at least 10 minutes three times a week to this practice.

Water Intake:

> Drink at least two liters of water per day, in small sips throughout the day. Add a crystal of Celtic or Himalayan salt to each glass to facilitate water access to every cell.

Laughter:

>Laughter has a relaxing effect on the colon. Children laugh up to 125 times a day; let's take inspiration from them to improve the health of our colon.

Vegetable Fibers:

>A high amount of fiber from vegetables not only aids the colon but also provides a lot of energy. There are no limits to vegetable consumption; it is important to consume them both raw and cooked.

Listen to the Body:

>Paying attention to the body's signals is crucial, especially when it comes to going to the bathroom. Responding promptly to such signals helps maintain a healthy colon.

The combination of these practices can promote colon stimulation and contribute to maintaining good intestinal health.

FOR GOOD LIVER FUNCTION

The liver is one of the most important organs in our body, performing various fundamental functions for health. The liver cleanses the blood of toxins, breaks down dead hemoglobin cells, regulates hormones, especially insulin, thus rebalancing blood glucose levels and the amount of energy available. Therefore, regularly purifying the liver is essential to enable it to perform all the "maintenance operations" that allow us to feel well.

There are herbs that stimulate liver healing and help keep it clean and healthy, especially bitter herbs. The liver is a repairable organ, so by stimulating and keeping the colon healthy and consuming the bitter herbs listed below, the liver will repair itself:

- Dandelion. It can be eaten fresh or as dried herb.
- Milk thistle.
- Gentian.
- Ginger.
- Artichoke.

Below, you will find two preparations for an effective liver detoxification.

Liver Cleanse

The Liver Cleanse is a powerful liver detoxification method. Follow these steps carefully to benefit from regenerative cleansing.

Required Ingredients:

1. One cup of fresh orange and lemon juice or grapefruit juice (the video uses one grapefruit and one lemon)
2. One cup of pure water
3. One clove of garlic
4. Half a teaspoon of chopped ginger
5. One tablespoon of olive oil

Procedure:

1. Preparation of Ingredients:
   - Get a cup of fresh citrus juice.
   - Measure a cup of pure water.
   - Chop the garlic clove and ginger.
2. Blending:
   - Put all the ingredients in the blender, excluding the olive oil.
   - Add the olive oil into the blender lid's designated hole to prevent liquid separation.
   - Blend until you get a homogeneous mixture.

3. Consumption:
   - Drink the freshly prepared mixture immediately.
   - Wait 15 minutes before moving on to the Liver Tea.
4. Considerations:
   - Using a high-power blender is recommended to avoid any lumps.

After completing this Liver Cleanse, proceed carefully with the Liver Tea procedure. Remember that detoxification is a beneficial process for liver health, and by regularly following these rituals, you can enjoy long-term benefits.

Liver Tea

Liver Tea, the second part of a recommended liver cleanse to promote liver health, is consumed after having the morning liver cleansing mixture. Following the instructions below, you will learn how to prepare this detoxifying beverage through a simple yet powerful recipe.

Required Ingredients:

1. Dandelion root
2. Licorice root
3. Gentian root
4. Milk thistle
5. Goldenseal

Procedure:

1. Preparing Dry Ingredients:
   - Use dried dandelion root.
   - Measure a quarter cup of licorice root.
   - For powdered ingredients (milk thistle and goldenseal), use two tablespoons of powder each.
2. Mixing:
   - Mix all the ingredients in a bowl until you achieve a homogeneous blend.
   - Store the mixture in a glass jar.
3. Tea Preparation:
   - Bring two cups of water to a boil in a stainless steel pot.
   - Add a tablespoon of the liver tea herb mixture.
   - Let it simmer for 15 minutes after boiling lightly.
4. Straining and Cooling:
   - Strain the tea to separate the herbs from the beverage.
   - Wait for the tea to cool before consumption.
5. Consumption:
   - Consume one or two teaspoons of the liver tea herb mixture per day, diluted in 16 ounces of water for each person.

After following this procedure, you'll be ready to experience the benefits of Liver Tea. It is recommended to consume healthy and detoxifying meals throughout the day to maximize results.

FOR GASTROINTESTINAL WELL-BEING

A healthy gastrointestinal system is an essential foundation for preserving the overall well-being of our body. The intestine, with its intricate network of functions, goes beyond mere digestion and nutrient absorption. It plays a vital role in various metabolic and immune activities, significantly contributing to the physiological balance of the organism. Intestinal health not only promotes proper food assimilation but also supports immune defense, metabolic regulation, and the maintenance of homeostasis, reflecting its crucial importance in keeping the body in harmony and vitality.

The thick mucosal wall of the gastrointestinal tract has four fundamental functions for the correct functioning of the intestine:

1. Handles the final breakdown of food.
2. Is responsible for food absorption.
3. Protects the blood from potential harmful pathogens.
4. Nourishes the small cells lining the gastrointestinal tract.

What damages this crucial wall:

- Excessive use of antibiotics.
- Excessive use of birth control pills.
- Excessive use of cortisone.
- Excessive use of ibuprofen or anti-inflammatories in general.

How to heal and repair the gastrointestinal tract:

1. Avoid these foods:
    - Hybridized wheat.
    - Dairy products.
    - Refined sugar.
    - Refined foods.
    - Meat.

2. Take these products:
    - Probiotics - Application: Take a probiotic supplement forty-five minutes before breakfast.
    - Aloe Vera and Red Elm.

3. Use "Digestive Powder" for severe cases:

    - Preparation:
        - 8 parts red elm.
        - 1 part myrrh.
        - 1 part goldenseal.
    - Mix everything together after grinding the herbs into powder.

    - Application:
        - One teaspoon in about half a glass of warm water.
        - For more severe cases, take 4 teaspoons per day, before each meal and the last one before bedtime.
        - Once the situation stabilizes, take the powder twice a day: in the morning and before bedtime in the evening.

- Once you feel well, stop taking the powder.

- Benefits:
  - Helps in severe cases of colitis.
  - Contributes to rebalancing the gastrointestinal tract.

4. Use Flax Seeds for constipation:

  - Preparation:
    - Place two teaspoons of whole flax seeds in a glass or bowl.
    - Pour boiling water over them and, if desired, a little orange juice.

  - Application:
    - The boiling water poured over the flax seeds releases the gel present in the flax seeds.
    - Drink the glass before going to bed.

  - Benefits:
    - Flax seeds, with their gel, act as a broom, helping to open the intestines.

HEALTHY PRACTICES

WATER, ITS USE, AND CELTIC SALT

Water, the second essential element for life after oxygen, plays a crucial role in human health. Sodium and potassium rank third and fourth, respectively, in importance for our bodies.

DAILY WATER REQUIREMENT

Throughout a day, the human body eliminates about 2 liters of water, and it is crucial to replenish this amount through the intake of pure water to maintain balance. Gradually increasing daily water intake is essential to accustom the body to this beneficial ritual. Only pure water can genuinely hydrate and cleanse the body. Beverages like coffee, orange juice, or sugary drinks fail to meet the body's real water needs and, in fact, contribute to dehydration.

NEGATIVE EFFECTS OF DEHYDRATION

Dehydration can lead to various negative effects, such as stomach ulcers, headaches, pancreatic dysfunction (with a risk of long-term diabetes), constipation, and high blood pressure. However, dehydration is often just part of a broader issue related to unhealthy lifestyles, such as excessive caffeine consumption, improper salt use, or a sedentary lifestyle.

TIPS FOR IDEAL WATER INTAKE:

• Outside of Meals:
  - Consume water away from meals. During meals, it is important not to flood the stomach with water. Drinking many glasses of water away from meals is necessary. If you are already hydrated when sitting down to eat, you won't feel the need to drink while eating. Therefore, it is a good habit to remember to drink half an hour before meals, so there is no need to do so while eating.
• Small Quantities and Sips:
  - Drink small amounts at a time, never a whole glass, just a sip or two, wait even just 5 minutes, and then another sip.
• Aim for 8/10 glasses of water a day, well-distributed throughout the day.
Accompanied by Sodium and Potassium:
  - Drink it accompanied by sodium and potassium, but we'll see this in the next paragraph!

WATER AND CELTIC SALT

In nature, we find the highest amount of sodium in seawater, along with 92 other minerals. Of these 92 minerals, about 30% are sodium, and about 50% are chloride.

Humans collect the first crystals of salt formed when water evaporates, bleach them, add aluminum, and thus produce table salt. It is dangerous because it contains only two very hard minerals that would need all the other minerals found in seawater to be softened and balanced.

The highest concentration of minerals in our cells is potassium, outside the cell, there is a higher concentration of sodium, normally they are balanced because there is a membrane between the inside and outside that contains sodium and potassium pumps that work to maintain a balance between them.

The problem arises when not enough fruits and vegetables are eaten, from which the body takes most of the potassium, and too much table salt is used to season every dish, every day. This way, sodium levels increase, and potassium levels decrease, and inside the cell, there is more sodium than there should be. The cell swells, and that's how high blood pressure begins.

To overcome this type of problem, in addition to changing one's diet, introducing plenty of fruits and vegetables, and drinking at least two liters of water a day, there is Celtic Salt.

Celtic salt is a salt from Brittany, France, and is hand-harvested using traditional methods. It contains 82 minerals in their balanced and harmonious form. Celtic salt, besides being a source of iodine, contains magnesium, indeed, it contains three types of magnesium. Magnesium is a water-hungry molecule. For this reason, Celtic salt always appears moist. Magnesium is a water-hungry molecule, precisely why it helps water enter the cell.

HOW TO TAKE CELTIC SALT

Just put a crystal of Celtic salt on the tongue, allowing the mucous membranes to absorb the minerals, especially magnesium. Subsequently, by drinking a glass of water, magnesium pulls water into the cells. This quick hydration method can be integrated whenever you drink water.

Drinking small sips of a glass of water with a crystal of Celtic salt not only helps maintain adequate hydration but also provides a healthy and effective way to regain energy, far surpassing the benefits of a cup of coffee mid-morning. For those with high blood pressure, starting with very small crystals is advisable. Alternatively, Himalayan salt, rich in 70-75 minerals, can be an excellent substitute for traditional table salt.

ORAL HYGIENE

PRACTICES FOR DENTAL AND ORAL HEALTH

Dental health is crucial for overall well-being, and adopting daily habits can significantly contribute to maintaining it.

INTERNAL FLUIDS:

Blood and lymph constantly nourish the teeth. A healthy life with fresh air, sunlight, physical exercise, and a nourishing diet helps maintain the quality of these fluids. Managing stress and embracing a spiritual dimension add further benefits.

EXTERNAL FLUID: SALIVA:

Saliva is essential for oral cleanliness. Avoiding harmful substances, going to bed early, and maintaining a healthy lifestyle contribute to maximizing the benefits of saliva.

RECOMMENDED PRACTICES FOR ORAL HYGIENE:

1. After meals: Adopt proper oral hygiene as a ritual. Rinsing with seawater or baking soda prevents plaque formation.
2. Dental floss: Use dental floss to remove unwanted residues.
3. Oil Pulling: This Ayurvedic practice involves rinsing the mouth with coconut oil for 15-20 minutes. Do not swallow the oil; spit it

out and rinse with warm water. Although benefits are claimed by proponents, scientific evidence is limited.

CONSISTENCY IS KEY:

Integrate these practices into your daily routine consistently. Regular rinsing and cleanings will have a positive impact on long-term dental health.

LONG-LASTING BENEFITS:

Cavity prevention, support for the natural healing of teeth, and reduced dental risks are long-term benefits. These practices can avoid costly dental interventions.

FINAL CONSIDERATIONS:

Avoid harmful foods and pay attention to the diet. Crunchy foods like apples can strengthen teeth, gums, and the jaw. With consistency, these habits can reduce the need for expensive dental procedures and preserve dental health over time.

PHYSICAL EXERCISE

THE IMPORTANCE OF DAILY EXERCISE

Daily life, in all its hustle and complexity, requires a well-oiled machine to cope with everyday challenges. This vital machine is our body, an extraordinary creation designed for constant activity. The importance of physical exercise in our daily living cannot be emphasized enough.

Physical exercise is the fuel that powers our internal engine. Every day, we are immersed in a whirlwind of activities: we work, move, take care of household chores, yet often, we neglect our bodily machine. As a result, our overall health may suffer, and the body can become sluggish and inefficient.

Our creator designed this machine to be in continuous motion. It is in the daily flow of activity that our body finds its inherent strength and vitality. When we neglect physical exercise, we disregard the original design of our bodily machine, and it may start showing signs of wear and tear.

Imagine your day as a dance, an intricate choreography of movements and actions. Without proper preparation, the dance becomes tiresome, and our internal machine begins to groan under pressure. On the other hand, when we engage in daily exercise, we tune into the natural symphony of our body.

Embarking on a path of regular physical activity doesn't necessarily mean committing to hours of strenuous training. Even small daily actions, like a brisk walk, a stretching session, or a quick home workout, can trigger the vitality our body desires.

Start viewing your body as a vital machine that requires constant maintenance. Daily exercise is not just a good practice; it is a necessity to stay aligned with our intrinsic nature. Take care of your bodily machine, activate your internal engine, and get ready to face the dance of life with strength and vitality.

HIIT: HIGH-INTENSITY INTERVAL TRAINING

When it comes to physical exercise, a key recommendation from experts is High-Intensity Interval Training (HIIT). This form of training has been recognized as one of the most effective methods to preserve muscle health and promote overall well-being.
The HIIT concept revolves around intervals of high-intensity physical activity alternated with periods of recovery or less intense activity. This approach engages the heart and lungs, significantly increasing heart rate and respiration.

The key to the success of HIIT lies in its ability to push the body beyond its limits for short periods, followed by a recovery period. This variation in intensity is what makes the training so effective in engaging different muscle groups and enhancing the cardiorespiratory system.

During a HIIT session, the body is pushed to a higher level of effort compared to traditional training. This additional stimulus is what triggers significant benefits for muscle and overall health. Increased heart rate not only improves cardiorespiratory capacity but also contributes to preserving muscle strength.

It's essential to highlight that HIIT can be adapted to each individual's needs. Whether running, cycling, or using an elliptical machine, the essence of high-intensity interval training remains the same: pushing the body to the maximum for a short time, followed by a recovery period. This dynamic approach to physical exercise proves to be a valuable ally in the challenge of maintaining and enhancing muscle health.

VARIETY OF OPTIONS

When it comes to physical exercise, the key to maintaining motivation and achieving tangible results lies in variety. There are several options for physical activity, each offering unique benefits for muscle and overall health.

Running: One of the most accessible and convenient activities is running. It's an excellent way to increase heart rate and engage numerous muscle groups. Even a short run can make a difference, especially when practiced regularly.

Stationary Bike: For those who prefer training in controlled environments, using a stationary bike can be an excellent choice.

This type of exercise reduces impact on the joints while effectively engaging leg muscles.

Rebounding Exercises (Trampoline): A surprising but equally effective option is rebounding, also known as trampoline workouts. This exercise involves the entire body, from head to toe, stimulating blood circulation and improving muscle strength.

Push-Up: A classic resistance exercise, push-ups are an effective way to strengthen the upper limbs and core. They can be adapted to different intensity levels, making them accessible to a wide range of people.

REBOUNDING

When it comes to duration and frequency, the key is consistency. Even short but regular exercises can lead to significant results. For example, a 20-minute run three times a week or a 15-minute rebounding session each day can make a difference in maintaining muscular health.

It's important to choose activities that are sustainable in the long term and that adapt to individual needs. Diversifying exercises not only maintains interest but also ensures that different muscle groups are engaged fairly, contributing to overall muscular health.

Rebounding, often overlooked, emerges as a precious gem in the world of physical exercise—a practice that not only defies gravity but also rekindles the body's vitality through a series of distinctive physical effects. Discovered for its effectiveness, rebounding offers an intriguing and beneficial history that goes beyond its simple appearance.

The practice of rebounding was originally unveiled by Albert Carter, a trampolinist from the '80s. Through his observation of the extraordinary physical abilities of his children, who grew up in a trampoline environment, Carter initiated research that led to the discovery of the surprising effectiveness of rebounding. This simple act of jumping on a trampoline became the foundation of a revolutionary exercise.

A 1979 NASA study describes the trampoline as the most efficient tool ever conceived by humans. Compared to other aerobic exercises, the elastic mat has a low impact on your body and can be practiced safely by anyone: it's perfect for all ages and fitness levels.

It's not just a game but a true sport, a fun and effective aerobic activity that allows you to optimize results by reducing workout times.

Jumping on the trampoline works the heart, tones the entire body, improves circulation, balance, and coordination. It's enjoyable and, unlike running, doesn't involve trauma to joints, ligaments, and muscles.

The trampoline, designed for rebounding, allows for zero-impact aerobic exercise, harnessing the training power of jumping while minimizing stress on the joints and the risk of microtraumas and injuries. This makes it suitable even for overweight individuals looking to get back in shape.

During a rebounding session, you can alternate various jumping rhythms to the beat of music (forward jumps, side jumps, spins), working on balance and functionally engaging the entire body.

The use of arms is also incorporated, with the added benefit of increasing heart rate and making the exercise even more effective. You can train both indoors and outdoors, whenever you have a few minutes, as the trampoline allows you to optimize results by reducing workout times.

Moreover, it's suitable for all fitness levels, as the intensity and duration of the workout can be adjusted according to individual needs. Additionally, jumping stimulates endorphins, benefiting not only the physique but also the mood!

There are aerobic rebounding exercises, performed with alternating feet, excellent from a cardiovascular perspective, and seated rebounding (with bounces on the buttocks), exceptional for strengthening the core (abdominals, and lower back).

The rebounding approach is not to consider the body as separate parts (muscles, bones, heart) but as a unified entity, comprised of different elements interacting to ensure maximum efficiency of movement.

Jumping on the elastic trampoline improves blood circulation and the capacity of the heart and lungs, while also allowing for comprehensive strengthening because all muscles—from abdominal to spinal—are involved in maintaining posture and interact to ensure maximum efficiency of movement.

In reality, it's bouncing, not jumping, whether standing or seated. Landing on the mat helps avoid impact with the ground and overloading the ankles, knees, and back. Unlike activities like running, the rebounder doesn't entail trauma to joints, ligaments, and muscles.

The rebounder ensures the same benefits as cardiovascular exercise, thus:

- Positively affects the respiratory and circulatory system.
- Stimulates breathing, oxygenating tissues better, involving every single cell in the body.
- Burns calories: in a 60-minute session, between 400 and 700/800 calories are burned, depending on the intensity of the workout, making it excellent for weight loss.
- Strengthens and tones leg and trunk muscles, which are engaged in jumping.
- The workout also enhances coordination—bouncing means moving legs, arms, head, back, and torso in harmony.
- Helps counteract water retention caused by poor fluid drainage in tissues because jumping stimulates the lymphatic system and facilitates venous return. This

happens because the muscle contraction accompanying the athletic motion of jumping allows for an upward push of blood, improving water reabsorption and reducing cellulite imperfections.

- Aids in preventing osteoporosis: numerous studies have highlighted that consistent training based on jumping promotes bone remineralization.
- Improves proprioception, balance, and coordination, with positive consequences for all actions normally performed in daily life.
- Is suitable for those with venous insufficiency and varicose veins, also strengthening pelvic floor muscles.

REBOUNDING AND STRESS

According to some studies, there is a close correlation between rebounding and stress. In particular, practicing this type of exercise on the elastic mat seems to allow the body to receive significant benefits, including eustress (or good stress). Relaxing and having fun while working to stay fit create an ideal situation for overall well-being, both physically and mentally.

The correlation with stress is determined by the effects these exercises have on the psyche. Being inherently enjoyable, they trigger the release of endorphins in the brain, substances known to instill a sense of general well-being. It can be asserted that rebounding generates good stress, helping the body regenerate not only from a physical but also a psychological perspective. The exercises are simple and accessible to everyone, especially as they can be done at home.

Anxiety or depression states are generated, in most cases, by negative stress. Long working days, daily problems, or challenging life moments are all sources of concern. The correlation between negative stress and certain subsequently defined psychosomatic illnesses was already demonstrated in the 1930s.

Rebounding serves as a natural remedy for stress, allowing individuals to have fun while performing the exercises. For example, it has been proven that a single session of jumping on the trampoline to music rhythm can generate a psychological well-being sensation lasting from 90 to 120 minutes after the workout.

Moreover, it aids in eliminating stress generated by adrenaline and other similar hormones, providing a sense of regained energy for those who practice it (excellent for combating depressive states). On a physical level, it also stimulates appetite and promotes a more peaceful rest.

Barbara O'Neill asserts: "Perhaps people age because they stop jumping."

RECOMMENDATION FOR A REBOUNDER IN EVERY HOME

In appreciating the versatility of the rebounder, awareness of its availability regardless of weather conditions emerges. Its constant presence, sheltered from atmospheric constraints, offers an unparalleled opportunity to improve physical and visual health in every season.

The invitation to seriously consider purchasing a rebounder for the home is motivated by its effectiveness and versatility. Beyond complex gym equipment, the rebounder stands out for its accessibility and ease of use. Its presence in limited spaces becomes a tangible opportunity for anyone wishing to incorporate physical exercise into their daily routine.

The emphasis on accessibility is not limited to practicality but also underscores the importance of investing in one's health. The rebounder, with its ability to engage the lymphatic system, improve balance, and optimize visual health, proves to be a valuable ally in promoting overall well-being.

In a context where space and weather conditions can limit workout options, the rebounder emerges as a versatile and accessible solution for everyone. Recommending it for every home not only suggests a shift in perspective on the practice of physical exercise but also encourages a choice that can make a difference in long-term health.

Investing in one's well-being doesn't have to be complicated or expensive. The timeless presence of the rebounder offers an accessible, effective, and enjoyable solution to improve physical and visual health. The final invitation is to embrace this opportunity, making the rebounder an essential element in every home aspiring to promote a healthy and active lifestyle.

ELESTIC MAT EXERCISES AND HOME CIRCUIT

Below is a cardiovascular program consisting of 7 exercises for a variable workout lasting between 10 and 35 minutes, depending on your fitness level.

For beginners: Perform each exercise for 30 seconds and repeat the circuit 3 times. Then increase the intensity by doing each exercise for 40 seconds and, finally, for one minute.
For those already trained: Perform each exercise for one minute, repeating the circuit 5 times.

1 – Side to Side:
Start with feet together on one side of the trampoline. Utilize the elastic force to jump, keeping feet together, shifting the body weight to the opposite side of the trampoline.
(Variant "Front and Back": Perform the same movement by moving forward and backward on the trampoline.)

2 – Jumping Jack:
Start standing with legs together, arms along the sides. Utilize the rebound to spread the legs, bringing the arms up, then close them and return to the starting position.

3 – Twist:

Start with legs together on the trampoline. Utilize the rebound to perform a twisting motion, moving the arms in the opposite direction of the knees and toes.

4 – Power Squat:

Start standing with legs slightly apart. Use the rebound to lower the body, lowering the center of gravity toward the trampoline, and spreading the legs more, as if performing a squat, then return to the starting position.

5 – Curl:

Start standing with legs apart. Utilize the trampoline's rebound to alternate flexing the legs, bringing the heel towards the buttocks.

6 – Knee Up:

Start with feet together. Utilize the rebound to alternately lift the knees, counterbalancing with the opposite arm.

7 – Split:

Start with legs apart, one foot in front of the other. Use the rebound to alternate the front leg, counterbalancing with the arm opposite to the leg.

Before engaging in any sports activity, it is always necessary to undergo a specialized evaluation to exclude pathologies, perhaps unrecognized or not very symptomatic, especially affecting the cardiopulmonary and musculoskeletal systems, which could worsen, even dangerously, with increased physical exercise.

INTEGRATED APPROACH TO HEALTH

NAVIGATING THE LAWS OF HEALTH

The importance of health, often referred to as an invaluable treasure, resonates in the wise words of Ellen White, illuminating the path to care for our greatest asset. A precious instruction that opens the doors to a deeper understanding of the laws of health, the foundations upon which we build our long-term well-being.

The laws of health, as outlined by White, serve as pillars on which our vitality stands. They are the guardians of our existence, the keys to unlocking a life of prosperity and vitality. Through our exploration of these laws, we embark on a journey undertaken by those who embrace self-care awareness.

- Pure air, a fundamental element, becomes our first travel companion. Through deep inhalation of uncontaminated air, we instill in our cells the vitality that only the element of pure air can confer. It is a dance between us and the surrounding environment, a symphony of oxygen that nourishes our being.

- The sun, the great architect of energy, plays a crucial role in our well-being. A warm embrace of its light nourishes not only the body but also the soul. Sun exposure is crucial for the production of vitamin D in the human body, an essential nutrient for bone health with significant benefits to the immune system and various physiological processes. The psychological well-being resulting from sun exposure is undeniable. Sunlight can positively influence mood, regulate circadian rhythms, and contribute to mental well-being and sleep. Sun exposure is also associated with a reduced risk of certain diseases, such as rickets in children and some skin conditions.

A brief daily exposure, especially during morning hours, is often considered beneficial without excessive risks related to prolonged exposure to more intense sunlight. Therefore, the need to find a balance between sun exposure to reap the benefits of vitamin D and protection from potential excessive exposure to harmful UV rays must be considered.

- Temperance, a balanced concept of moderation, emerges as a valuable guide among the laws of health. It is the key to avoiding harmful extremes and embracing a lifestyle that nurtures without excess or deprivation. A harmonious dance between what we give our bodies and what our bodies truly need.

The goal is to maintain a balanced and varied diet, avoiding nutritional excesses or deficiencies. However, this approach extends beyond nutrition, incorporating balanced lifestyle habits such as moderate alcohol consumption, avoiding smoking, and maintaining an active and balanced lifestyle. Balancing the pleasure derived from dietary choices and lifestyle habits with the need to preserve long-term health is essential. Nutritional education becomes crucial in this context, promoting awareness of dietary choices as an integral part of temperance. In summary, temperance encourages a comprehensive approach that promotes a balanced lifestyle, without harmful excesses and with respect for long-term health.

- Rest, often overlooked in the hustle of modern life, becomes a precious gem on our journey. It is during rejuvenating sleep that our body renews itself, preparing for the challenges of the next day. Homage to rest becomes an investment in our long-term well-being.

- Exercise, a practice celebrated for centuries, proves to be a timeless law of health. Through mindful movement, we shape not only our bodies but also our minds. It is an act of gratitude for the gift of vitality, an ode to the strength that resides in each of us.

- A proper diet, an essential chapter in our exploration, teaches us that what we put into our bodies has a lasting impact on our health. It's a celebration of foods that nourish and support, a conscious choice for prosperity and well-being.
An in-depth look at crucial themes for health and wellness cannot overlook the Glycemic Index of Foods, the speed at which different foods can influence blood sugar levels, assessed through the Glycemic Index. Red fruits, such as cherries, are known for their low Glycemic Index, approximately around 25. Grapefruit is mentioned as another low Glycemic Index option, with a value of about 24. Sugar, whether white, brown, or cane, has a Glycemic Index of 59, ranking higher than many fruits. Surprisingly, white bread, made with refined flour, shows a GI of 69, positioning it above sugar.

The effects of coffee and caffeine on the nervous system also merit consideration. Caffeine plays a fundamental role by interfering with adenosine, a neurotransmitter that acts as a brake in the nervous system. Ingesting caffeine reduces adenosine levels, creating a sensation of a missing brake and increasing stimulation.

Another interesting aspect concerns the influence of caffeine on acetylcholine, a crucial neurotransmitter for brain functions. This impact could manifest through effects on concentration and cognitive functions, adding a significant element to caffeine consumption. A third point of reflection focuses on the relationship between caffeine and dopamine, a neurotransmitter linked to feelings of reward and happiness. The increase in dopamine could explain the common perception of coffee as a stimulant and energizer, providing insight into the connection between caffeine and psychological well-being. Examining these aspects reveals an intricate connection between caffeine and neurological mechanisms, highlighting how coffee consumption can affect various levels of nervous system regulation.

The use of water, often considered simple in its essence, becomes an elixir of life in the laws of health. Special attention should be given to hydration and the promotion of health through water. Water is an essential element for the health and well-being of the body, and the proper use of this vital liquid is considered an integral part of practices to maintain a healthy lifestyle. It's important to drink a sufficient amount of high-quality water to

127

keep the body well-hydrated because hydration is a key component in the broader context of health. Water plays a crucial role in the fundamental biological processes of the body, including digestion, elimination of toxins, and maintenance of water balance.

- Trust in divine power, the last but not least important law, becomes the guiding thread that intertwines all others. Establishing a spiritual connection and nurturing faith in a higher power can promote health and well-being. Recognizing and cultivating the spiritual element in a person's life can be immensely helpful, as health encompasses not only the physical body but also the spiritual dimension of being. Daily spiritual practices, such as prayer, meditation, or other forms of spiritual reflection, can contribute to strengthening the connection with a divine power and bring psychological and physical benefits derived from trust in a higher power, such as increased serenity, reduced stress, and overall emotional well-being. It's crucial to emphasize that the approach aims not to promote a specific religious tradition but rather encourages individuals to find a spiritual connection that resonates with their personal understanding.

Through understanding and adherence to these laws of health, we plant the seeds for a life of prosperity and vitality. This journey into the laws of health becomes a commitment to a life that reflects awareness, care, and love for ourselves.

IN-DEPTH ON PURE AIR

The air we breathe is the first step in the choreography of health, an invisible dance that connects us to the very vitality of life. Navigating the intricacies of pure air, the first law of health, opens the doors to a world of enduring well-being.

Vital Importance of Pure Air:
Pure air is not merely an environmental element but an essential nourishment for our body and mind. With every breath, we immerse ourselves in an inexhaustible source of vital energy. It forms the foundation upon which our health stands, an element often taken for granted in the hustle of modern life.

The Magic of Negative Ions:
At the heart of this symphony of pure air are negative ions, small allies that carry a baggage of benefits. Negative ions, abundant in natural environments like forests, waterfalls, and ocean waves, are like little messengers of freshness. They stimulate our body and mind, improving mood and reducing stress.

The Difference between Positive and Negative Ions:
It is crucial to understand the difference between positive and negative ions. While negative ions promote health and well-being, positive ions, often dominant in urban areas, can have negative effects. Their presence is associated with increased stress, fatigue, and tension. Our daily hustle can expose us to an excess of positive ions, challenging our internal balance.

Abundant Sources of Negative Ions:

To immerse oneself in the beneficial atmosphere of negative ions, it is essential to know their sources. Thunderstorms, with their electric spectacle, generate a cascade of negative ions. Ocean waves breaking, cascading waterfalls, and forests, especially those inhabited by pine trees, are rich sanctuaries of these small health allies.

Negative Impact of Positive Ions:

In urban areas, positive ions can proliferate, creating an imbalance in the delicate equilibrium of our well-being. Sources of electromagnetic pollution and modern electronics contribute to the generation and accumulation of positive ions, putting our long-term health at risk.

Vital Oxygen: The Fuel of Life

On the stage of health, oxygen emerges as the undisputed protagonist, the fuel that powers the uninterrupted dance of life within our bodies. Let's explore the physiological enchantment of oxygen, revealing its profound and vital impact.

Breath of Life:

Oxygen is the breath of life, an invisible force that sustains every beat of our heart and every step of our journey. When we inhale, we welcome into our cells an elixir of life that fuels essential processes for our well-being.

Symptoms of Hypoxemia:

The lack of oxygen, known as hypoxia, can manifest through subtle symptoms that draw attention from our bodies. Dizziness, fatigue, and confusion are signals that our body sends when the oxygen levels reach critical levels. Listening to these signals is crucial to intervene and restore balance.

The Heart of Energy:

In addition to its role in ensuring proper brain function, oxygen plays a central role in energy production. The cells of our bodies, through complex processes like cellular respiration, transform oxygen into usable energy. It's the engine that powers every action, from a simple blink of an eye to a strenuous run.

Cellular Processes:

Our cells, the fundamental elements of our being, depend on oxygen to perform their vital tasks. From cellular repair processes to immune defense, oxygen is the key that unlocks the potential of our cells. Its presence guarantees optimal functioning of the mechanisms that make up the fabric of life.

In this act of our exploration of the laws of health, we highlight the critical role of oxygen. It is the invisible thread that connects every aspect of our being, an essential treasure often overlooked in the hustle of modern life. Let us consciously breathe, embracing the power of oxygen as the foundation on which our vitality rests.

CONCLUSION

This book is an invitation to explore the transformative power of natural remedies, inspired by the precious teachings of Barbara O'Neill. Each page is woven with care, offering not only practical advice but also a refuge of wisdom and awareness.

The proposed remedies, rooted in nature, become a bridge between ancient knowledge and our present well-being. Through the lens of natural health, we learn to understand the language of our bodies, to respect the rhythm of nature, and to cultivate a deep connection with the world around us.

In this tribute to Barbara, we celebrate her dedication to a life in harmony with nature. Every reader is invited to reap the fruits of this knowledge, to explore their own healing journey, and to embrace a lifestyle that resonates with natural health.

May "Home Remedies" be a faithful companion on your journey to well-being. Through the principles of natural health, we can rediscover the healing power that resides within us and embrace a holistic approach to health, in harmony with Barbara O'Neill's vision.

Thank you for sharing this journey with us. May the light of natural health continue to illuminate your path, offering nourishment and balance at every step.

Thank you for purchasing this book!

If you enjoyed it, please leave a brief review. Your feedback is important to us and will help other readers decide whether to read the book too.
For a small company like us, getting reviews means a lot to us.
We can't THANK YOU enough for this!

About PrimeInsight Press

At PrimeInsight Press, our story begins as a passionate small team with a belief: knowledge, when shared with passion, can create positive change. We have dedicated ourselves to creating authentic, and professional guides, also paying special attention to their high-quality, engaging interior design.
We believe that every book is an opportunity to touch hearts and empower minds. Through the pages of our books, we hope to inspire you to dream and provide you with the tools to bring those dreams to life.
Join us at PrimeInsight Press, and together, transform your journey of growth, one page at a time.

Important Notice

We take customer suggestions seriously. If you have any, please write to: primeinsightpress@gmail.com and include the book's title in the email subject.

SCAN the QR Code
to Enjoy the Audiobook

Made in the USA
Monee, IL
11 February 2024

53344364R00075